LOW FODMAP DIET COOKBOOK FOR BEGINNERS

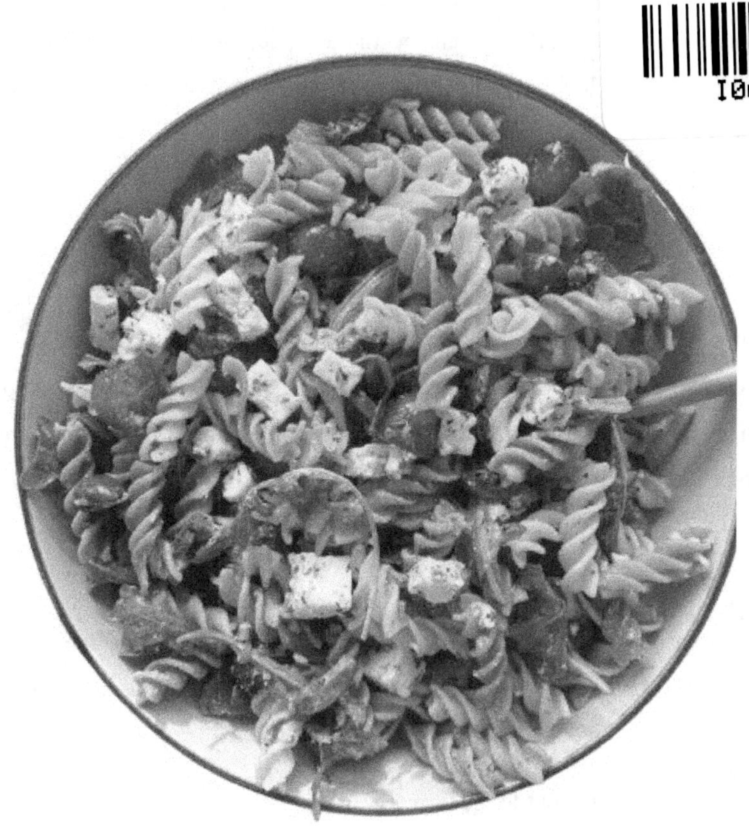

LYSANDRA QUINN

Copyright © 2023 by Lysandra Quinn
All rights reserved.

DISCLAIMER

Contact the Author

Thank you for reading my book! I would love to hear from you, whether you have feedback, questions, or just want to share your thoughts. Your feedback means a lot to me and helps me improve as a writer.

Please don't hesitate to reach out to me through

contactmelysandraquinn@gmail.com

I look forward to connecting with my readers and appreciate your support in this literary journey. Your thoughts and comments are valuable to me.

TABLE OF CONTENTS

INTRODUCTION

In the quiet corners of our lives, where health meets flavour, there exists a tapestry woven with the threads of shared experiences and the profound impact of simple, yet transformative recipes. It's a narrative that I stumbled upon not in a sterile lab but in the warm embrace of friendship and the resilient spirit of my dear friend, Elaine.

Elaine, a vivacious soul with a penchant for life's pleasures, found herself entangled in the complexities of digestive discomfort. Countless cookbooks had passed through her hands like fleeting seasons, each promising relief, yet none delivering the solace she sought. In her quest for culinary solutions, she traversed a labyrinth of ingredients and methods, only to find herself standing at the crossroads of frustration and despair.

As a seasoned dietitian, I had spent years immersed in the world of nutrition, navigating the ebbs and flows of dietary trends. But it was Elaine's journey that became my catalyst for delving into the intricate realm of the Low FODMAP diet. Witnessing her struggles ignited a fire within me, compelling me to channel my expertise into crafting a collection of recipes that would not merely satiate hunger but also nurture gut health.

It began with a simple gesture—a binder filled with meticulously researched and thoughtfully curated Low FODMAP recipes. I handed it to Elaine, not as a dietician, but as a friend eager to alleviate her discomfort. Little did I know that this humble offering would set in motion a culinary odyssey, transforming Elaine's life and inspiring the creation of this cookbook.

As the pages of this cookbook unfold, each recipe is infused with the passion and dedication born from Elaine's journey. They are not just a compilation of ingredients and instructions; they are an invitation to embark on a transformative adventure—one that transcends the realm of mere sustenance and delves deep into the art of healing through nourishment.

Now, let me take you on a journey through these pages, where the aroma of spices mingles with the essence of triumph, and the Flavors dance in harmony with the rhythm of restored well-being. Before you dive into the heart of this cookbook, consider the questions that might resonate with your own experiences:

Have you ever felt the frustration of trying countless diets, only to find yourself back at square one?

Do you yearn for a cookbook that not only tantalizes your taste buds but also addresses the unique needs of your digestive system?

Can you envision a life where meals are not just about filling your stomach but about nourishing your body and soul?

Have you ever longed for a community that understands the challenges of embracing dietary changes and supports you every step of the way?

Are you ready to unlock the potential of a diet that goes beyond the superficial and delves into the profound impact it can have on your overall well-being?

If any of these questions resonate with you, then you're not just holding a cookbook; you're cradling a lifeline—a guide that transcends the boundaries of conventional culinary literature and invites you to join a community of individuals who have walked the path of digestive resilience.

In the chapters that follow, you'll find not just recipes but stories—stories of hope, resilience, and the unwavering belief that a happy gut leads to a happy life. As you embark on this gastronomic adventure, may the dishes you create become more than just meals; may they become the building blocks of your own journey towards a deliciously happy and healthy life.

So, with anticipation in your heart and a hunger for more than just food, let's dive into the world of " Low FODMAP Diet Cookbook for Beginners."

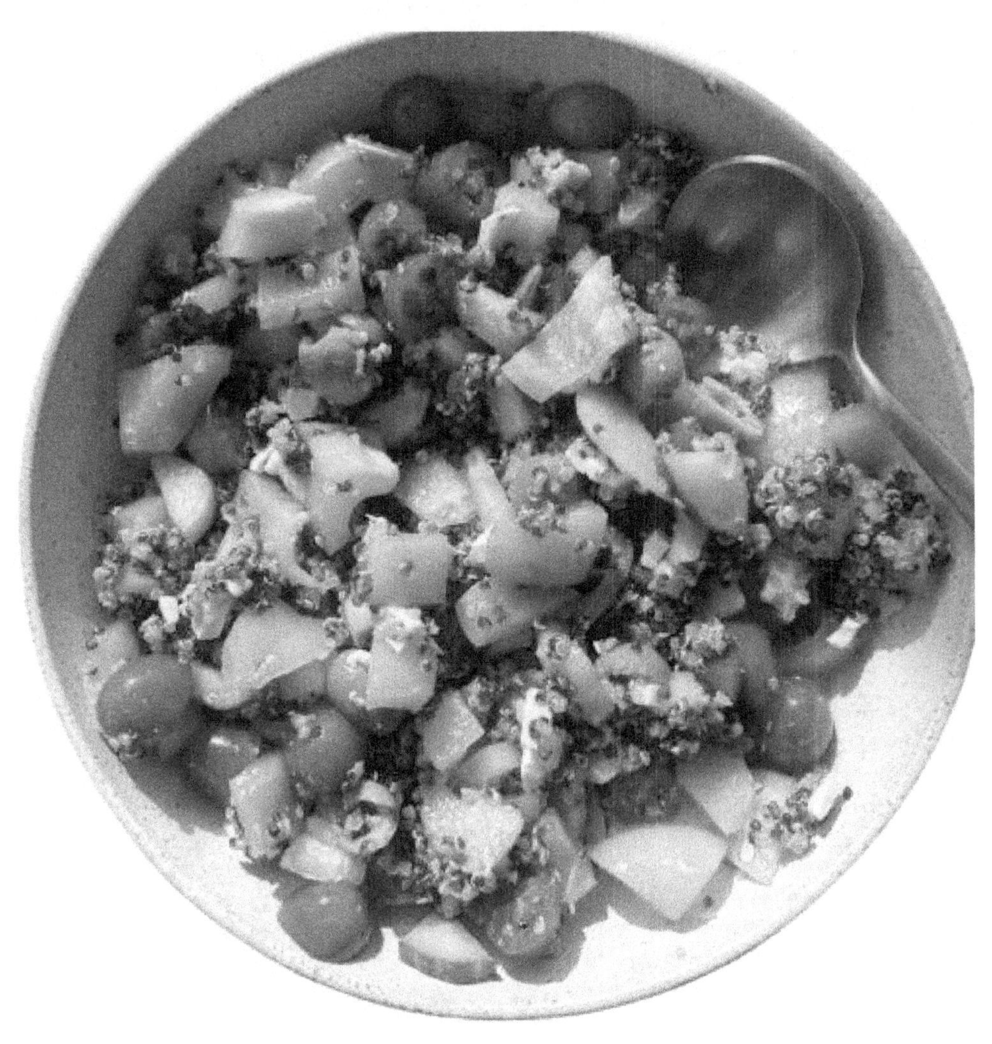

CHAPTER 1

UNDERSTANDING FODMAPS

The Low FODMAP lifestyle has gained increasing attention in recent years as a potential solution for managing digestive discomfort. FODMAPs, short for Fermentable Oligosaccharides, Disaccharides, Monosaccharides, and Polyols, are a group of carbohydrates that can cause digestive issues in susceptible individuals. In this exploration, we will unveil the mystery of FODMAPs, understand how they impact digestive health, and delve into the science behind the Low FODMAP Diet.

Unveiling the Mystery of FODMAPs:

FODMAPs are a diverse group of carbohydrates found in various foods, including fruits, vegetables, grains, and dairy products. The complexity lies in their fermentable nature, which means they can be rapidly fermented by gut bacteria, leading to the production of gas and other byproducts. For individuals with sensitive digestive systems, this fermentation process can result in symptoms such as bloating, gas, abdominal pain, and altered bowel habits.

How FODMAPs Impact Your Digestive Health:

Understanding the impact of FODMAPs on digestive health is crucial for those seeking relief from gastrointestinal issues. When FODMAPs are poorly absorbed in the small intestine, they travel to the colon where they become a feast for gut bacteria. This fermentation process can lead to the production of gases, causing distension and discomfort. Moreover, FODMAPs draw water into the intestines, potentially contributing to diarrhea in some individuals.

The Science Behind the Low FODMAP Diet:

The Low FODMAP Diet, developed by researchers at Monash University, aims to reduce the intake of fermentable carbohydrates to alleviate digestive symptoms. The diet involves three main phases: restriction, reintroduction, and personalization. During the restriction phase, high FODMAP foods are eliminated to provide relief. The reintroduction phase involves systematically reintroducing FODMAP groups to identify specific triggers for each individual. Finally, the personalization phase establishes a sustainable, personalized diet that minimizes symptoms.

CHAPTER 2

DELICIOUSLY DIGESTIBLE

BREAKFASTS

Banana and Blueberry Quinoa Porridge

Cooking Time: 15 minutes

Servings: 2

Ingredients:

- 1 cup quinoa flakes
- 1 ripe banana, mashed.
- 1/2 cup blueberries
- 2 cups lactose-free milk
- 1 tablespoon maple syrup (optional)
- 1 tablespoon chopped walnuts (optional)

Instructions:

1. In a saucepan, combine quinoa flakes, mashed banana, blueberries, and lactose-free milk.
2. Cook over medium heat, stirring frequently, until the porridge thickens (about 10-12 minutes).
3. Sweeten with maple syrup if desired and top with chopped walnuts.
4. Serve warmly.

Nutritional Information (per serving):

Calories: 350, Protein: 12g, Carbohydrates: 60g, Fiber: 7g, Fat: 8g

Spinach and Feta Omelet

Cooking Time: 10 minutes

Servings: 1

Ingredients:

- 3 large eggs
- 1/2 cup fresh spinach, chopped.
- 2 tablespoons feta cheese, crumbled.
- Salt and pepper to taste
- 1 tablespoon olive oil

Instructions:

1. Whisk eggs in a bowl and season with salt and pepper.
2. Heat olive oil in a non-stick pan over medium heat.
3. Add chopped spinach to the pan and sauté until wilted.
4. Pour the whisked eggs over the spinach, sprinkle with feta, and cook until set.
5. Fold the omelette in half and serve.

Nutritional Information:

Calories: 350, Protein: 20g, Carbohydrates: 4g, Fat: 28g

Chia Seed Pudding with Berries

Prep Time: 5 minutes (+overnight soaking)

Servings: 2

Ingredients:

- 1/4 cup chia seeds
- 1 cup lactose-free milk
- 1 tablespoon maple syrup
- 1/2 teaspoon vanilla extract
- Mixed berries for topping

Instructions:

1. In a bowl, mix chia seeds, milk, maple syrup, and vanilla extract.
2. Stir well, cover, and refrigerate overnight.
3. In the morning, stir the pudding and top with mixed berries.

Nutritional Information (per serving):

Calories: 180, Protein: 6g, Carbohydrates: 20g, Fiber: 10g, Fat: 8g

Turkey and Vegetable Breakfast Skillet

Cooking Time: 20 minutes

Servings: 2

Ingredients:

- 1/2 lb ground turkey
- 1 bell pepper, diced.
- 1 zucchini, diced.
- 1 teaspoon garlic-infused olive oil
- Salt and pepper to taste
- 4 eggs

Instructions:

1. In a skillet, cook ground turkey in garlic-infused olive oil until browned.
2. Add diced bell pepper and zucchini and cook until vegetables are tender.
3. Season with salt and pepper.
4. Make four wells in the mixture and crack an egg into each.
5. Cover and cook until eggs are done to your liking.

Nutritional Information (per serving):

Calories: 320, Protein: 28g, Carbohydrates: 8g, Fat: 18g

Peanut Butter Banana Smoothie

Prep Time: 5 minutes

Servings: 1

Ingredients:

- 1 ripe banana
- 1 tablespoon peanut butter
- 1 cup lactose-free yogurt
- 1/2 cup ice cubes
- 1 tablespoon chia seeds (optional)

Instructions:

1. Blend banana, peanut butter, lactose-free yogurt, and ice cubes until smooth.
2. Pour into a glass, top with chia seeds if desired, and enjoy.

Nutritional Information:

Calories: 350, Protein: 15g, Carbohydrates: 40g, Fat: 15g

Blueberry Almond Overnight Oats

Prep Time: 5 minutes (+overnight soaking)

Servings: 2

Ingredients:

- 1 cup rolled oats.
- 1 cup lactose-free milk
- 1/2 cup blueberries
- 2 tablespoons almond butter
- 1 tablespoon maple syrup

Instructions:

1. In a jar, combine oats, milk, blueberries, almond butter, and maple syrup.
2. Stir well, cover, and refrigerate overnight.
3. In the morning, give it a good stir and enjoy.

Nutritional Information (per serving):

Calories: 380, Protein: 12g, Carbohydrates: 50g, Fiber: 8g, Fat: 16g

Low FODMAP Breakfast Burrito

Cooking Time: 15 minutes

Servings: 2

Ingredients:

- 4 corn tortillas
- 4 eggs, scrambled.
- 1 cup spinach, chopped.
- 1/2 cup cherry tomatoes, halved.
- 1/4 cup lactose-free cheese, shredded.
- Salsa for topping

Instructions:

1. Warm tortillas in a dry skillet.
2. Fill each tortilla with scrambled eggs, chopped spinach, tomatoes, and cheese.
3. Roll into burritos and top with salsa.

Nutritional Information (per serving):

Calories: 320, Protein: 18g, Carbohydrates: 30g, Fat: 14g

Cinnamon Maple Pecan Granola Parfait

Prep Time: 10 minutes

Servings: 2

Ingredients:

- 1 cup low FODMAP granola
- 1 cup lactose-free yogurt
- 1/4 cup pecans, chopped.
- 1 tablespoon maple syrup
- 1/2 teaspoon ground cinnamon

Instructions:

1. In serving glasses, layer granola, yogurt, and chopped pecans.
2. Drizzle with maple syrup and sprinkle with ground cinnamon.
3. Repeat the layers and enjoy.

Nutritional Information (per serving):

Calories: 400, Protein: 12g, Carbohydrates: 45g, Fiber: 6g, Fat: 20g

Smoked Salmon and Avocado Toast

Cooking Time: 10 minutes

Servings: 2

Ingredients:

- 4 slices gluten-free bread
- 1 avocado, sliced.
- 4 oz smoked salmon
- 1 tablespoon lemon juice
- Chives for garnish

Instructions:

1. Toast the gluten-free bread slices.
2. Top each slice with sliced avocado and smoked salmon.
3. Drizzle with lemon juice and garnish with chives.

Nutritional Information (per serving):

Calories: 320, Protein: 18g, Carbohydrates: 20g, Fat: 18g

Greek Yogurt and Berry Parfait

Prep Time: 10 minutes

Servings: 2

Ingredients:

- 2 cups lactose-free Greek yogurt
- 1 cup mixed berries (strawberries, blueberries, raspberries)
- 1/4 cup low FODMAP granola
- 1 tablespoon honey (optional)

Instructions:

1. In serving glasses, layer Greek yogurt, mixed berries, and granola.
2. Repeat the layers.
3. Drizzle with honey if desired.

Nutritional Information (per serving):

Calories: 250, Protein: 15g, Carbohydrates: 30g, Fat: 8g

CHAPTER 3

LUNCHTIME BLISS: GUT-FRIENDLY MIDDAY MEALS

Grilled Chicken Salad with Citrus Dressing

Cooking Time: 20 minutes

Servings: 2

Ingredients:

- 2 boneless, skinless chicken breasts
- Mixed salad greens
- 1 orange peeled and segmented.
- 1/4 cup sliced cucumber.
- 1 tablespoon olive oil
- 1 tablespoon balsamic vinegar
- Salt and pepper to taste

Instructions:

1. Season chicken breasts with salt and pepper, then grill until fully cooked.
2. In a bowl, toss salad greens, orange segments, and sliced cucumber.
3. Slice grilled chicken and place on top of the salad.
4. Whisk together olive oil and balsamic vinegar for the dressing.
5. Drizzle dressing over the salad and serve.

Nutritional Information (per serving):

Calories: 350, Protein: 30g, Carbohydrates: 15g, Fat: 18g

Quinoa and Roasted Vegetable Bowl

Cooking Time: 25 minutes

Servings: 2

Ingredients:

- 1 cup cooked quinoa
- Assorted low FODMAP roasted vegetables (zucchini, bell peppers, cherry tomatoes)
- 1/4 cup feta cheese, crumbled.
- Fresh basil leaves for garnish.
- Olive oil for drizzling

Instructions:

1. Cook quinoa according to package instructions.
2. Roast vegetables in olive oil until tender.
3. In a bowl, combine quinoa, roasted vegetables, and crumbled feta.
4. Drizzle with olive oil, garnish with fresh basil, and serve.

Nutritional Information (per serving):

Calories: 380, Protein: 12g, Carbohydrates: 45g, Fat: 18g

Turkey and Cranberry Wrap

Prep Time: 15 minutes

Servings: 2

Ingredients:

- 4 gluten-free tortillas
- 1/2 lb sliced turkey.
- 1/4 cup cranberry sauce
- 1 cup spinach leaves
- 1/4 cup lactose-free cheese, shredded.

Instructions:

1. Lay out tortillas and distribute turkey slices evenly.
2. Spread cranberry sauce over the turkey.
3. Top with spinach leaves and shredded lactose-free cheese.
4. Roll into wraps and slice in half before serving.

Nutritional Information (per serving):

Calories: 320, Protein: 18g, Carbohydrates: 30g, Fat: 15g

Salmon and Quinoa Stuffed Bell Peppers

Cooking Time: 30 minutes

Servings: 2

Ingredients:

- 2 bell peppers halved, and seeds removed.
- 1/2 lb cooked salmon, flaked.
- 1 cup cooked quinoa
- 1/4 cup cherry tomatoes, halved.
- Fresh dill for garnish
- Lemon wedges for serving.

Instructions:

1. Preheat oven to 375°F (190°C).
2. In a bowl, mix flaked salmon, cooked quinoa, and cherry tomatoes.
3. Stuff bell peppers with the salmon mixture.
4. Bake for 20-25 minutes or until peppers are tender.
5. Garnish with fresh dill and serve with lemon wedges.

Nutritional Information (per serving):

Calories: 400, Protein: 25g, Carbohydrates: 30g, Fat: 20g

Eggplant and Tomato Caprese Stack

Cooking Time: 15 minutes

Servings: 2

Ingredients:

- 1 large eggplant, sliced.
- 2 tomatoes, sliced.
- 1/2 cup fresh mozzarella, sliced.
- Fresh basil leaves
- Balsamic glaze for drizzling

Instructions:

1. Grill or roast eggplant slices until tender.
2. Assemble stacks by layering eggplant, tomato, and mozzarella.
3. Top each stack with fresh basil leaves.
4. Drizzle with balsamic glaze and serve.

Nutritional Information (per serving):

Calories: 280, Protein: 15g, Carbohydrates: 20g, Fat: 15g

Shrimp and Vegetable Stir-Fry

Cooking Time: 20 minutes

Servings: 2

Ingredients:

- 1/2 lb shrimp, peeled and deveined.
- Assorted low FODMAP stir-fry vegetables (bell peppers, zucchini, carrots)
- 2 tablespoons soy sauce (use gluten-free if needed)
- 1 tablespoon sesame oil
- 1 tablespoon green onion, green parts only, chopped (optional)

Instructions:

1. Heat sesame oil in a wok or skillet.
2. Add shrimp and stir-fry until pink and opaque.
3. Add vegetables and continue stir-frying until tender.
4. Pour in soy sauce and toss to combine.
5. Garnish with chopped green onion if desired and serve.

Nutritional Information (per serving):

Calories: 300, Protein: 25g, Carbohydrates: 15g, Fat: 15g

Lemon Dill Chicken Salad Lettuce Wraps

Prep Time: 15 minutes

Servings: 2

Ingredients:

- 1 cup cooked chicken, shredded.
- 2 tablespoons mayonnaise
- 1 tablespoon Dijon mustard
- 1 tablespoon fresh dill, chopped.
- Salt and pepper to taste
- Large lettuce leaves for wrapping.

Instructions:

1. In a bowl, mix shredded chicken, mayonnaise, Dijon mustard, and chopped dill.
2. Season with salt and pepper to taste.
3. Spoon chicken salad onto lettuce leaves and wrap.
4. Secure with toothpicks if needed and serve.

Nutritional Information (per serving):

Calories: 250, Protein: 20g, Carbohydrates: 5g, Fat: 16g

Tomato Basil Zoodle Bowl

Cooking Time: 15 minutes

Servings: 2

Ingredients:

- 2 zucchinis, spiralized into noodles
- 1 cup cherry tomatoes, halved.
- 2 tablespoons olive oil
- 1/4 cup fresh basil, chopped.
- Parmesan cheese, grated (optional)

Instructions:

1. Heat olive oil in a pan and sauté zucchini noodles until just tender.
2. Add cherry tomatoes and cook for an additional 2-3 minutes.
3. Stir in chopped fresh basil.
4. Serve topped with grated Parmesan if desired.

Nutritional Information (per serving):

Calories: 200, Protein: 5g, Carbohydrates: 10g, Fat: 15g

Low FODMAP Tuna Salad Stuffed Avocado

Prep Time: 10 minutes

Servings: 2

Ingredients:

- 2 ripe avocados halved and pitted.
- 1 can (5 oz) tuna, drained
- 2 tablespoons mayonnaise
- 1 tablespoon lemon juice
- Salt and pepper to taste

Instructions:

1. In a bowl, mix tuna, mayonnaise, and lemon juice.
2. Season with salt and pepper to taste.
3. Spoon tuna salad into avocado halves.
4. Serve as a refreshing and filling salad.

Nutritional Information (per serving):

Calories: 300, Protein: 15g, Carbohydrates: 10g, Fat: 25g

Mediterranean Quinoa Bowl

Cooking Time: 20 minutes

Servings: 2

Ingredients:

- 1 cup cooked quinoa
- 1/2 cup cucumber, diced.
- 1/2 cup cherry tomatoes, halved.
- 1/4 cup Kalamata olives, sliced.
- 2 tablespoons feta cheese, crumbled.
- 1 tablespoon olive oil
- Fresh oregano for garnish

Instructions:

1. In a bowl, combine cooked quinoa, diced cucumber, cherry tomatoes, olives, and crumbled feta.
2. Drizzle with olive oil and toss to combine.
3. Garnish with fresh oregano and serve.

Nutritional Information (per serving):

Calories: 350, Protein: 10g, Carbohydrates: 45g, Fat: 15g

CHAPTER 3

DINNER DELIGHTS: SAVORY CREATIONS FOR A CALM BELLY

Grilled Lemon Herb Chicken

Cooking Time: 25 minutes

Servings: 4

Ingredients:

- 4 boneless, skinless chicken breasts
- 2 tablespoons olive oil
- 1 lemon, juiced.
- 1 teaspoon dried oregano
- 1 teaspoon dried thyme
- Salt and pepper to taste

Instructions:

1. Preheat the grill to medium-high heat.
2. In a bowl, mix olive oil, lemon juice, oregano, thyme, salt, and pepper.
3. Brush the chicken breasts with the marinade.
4. Grill for 6-8 minutes per side or until fully cooked.
5. Serve with your favorite low FODMAP side dishes.

Nutritional Information (per serving):

Calories: 250, Protein: 30g, Carbohydrates: 1g, Fat: 13g

Baked Salmon with Dill and Lemon

Cooking Time: 20 minutes

Servings: 4

Ingredients:

- 4 salmon fillets
- 2 tablespoons fresh dill, chopped.
- 1 lemon, sliced.
- 2 tablespoons olive oil
- Salt and pepper to taste

Instructions:

1. Preheat the oven to 400°F (200°C).
2. Place salmon fillets on a baking sheet.
3. Drizzle with olive oil and season with salt, pepper, and chopped dill.
4. Top each fillet with lemon slices.
5. Bake for 15-20 minutes or until salmon flakes easily with a fork.

Nutritional Information (per serving):

Calories: 300, Protein: 25g, Carbohydrates: 0g, Fat: 20g

Low FODMAP Beef and Vegetable Stir-Fry

Cooking Time: 20 minutes

Servings: 4

Ingredients:

- 1 lb beef sirloin, thinly sliced.
- Assorted low FODMAP stir-fry vegetables (bell peppers, bok choy, carrots)
- 2 tablespoons soy sauce (use gluten-free if needed)
- 1 tablespoon garlic-infused olive oil
- Sesame seeds for garnish (optional)

Instructions:

1. Heat garlic-infused olive oil in a wok or skillet.
2. Add sliced beef and stir-fry until browned.
3. Add vegetables and continue stir-frying until tender.
4. Pour in soy sauce and toss to combine.
5. Garnish with sesame seeds if desired and serve.

Nutritional Information (per serving):

Calories: 350, Protein: 30g, Carbohydrates: 10g, Fat: 20g

Lemon Garlic Shrimp and Zucchini Noodles

Cooking Time: 15 minutes

Servings: 2

Ingredients:

- 1/2 lb shrimp, peeled and deveined.
- 2 zucchinis, spiralized into noodles
- 2 tablespoons olive oil
- 2 cloves garlic, minced.
- 1 lemon, juiced.
- Salt and pepper to taste
- Fresh parsley for garnish

Instructions:

1. Heat olive oil in a pan and sauté minced garlic until fragrant.
2. Add shrimp and cook until pink and opaque.
3. Add zucchini noodles and cook for 2-3 minutes.
4. Drizzle with lemon juice, season with salt and pepper, and garnish with fresh parsley.

Nutritional Information (per serving):

Calories: 250, Protein: 20g, Carbohydrates: 10g, Fat: 15g

Quinoa Stuffed Bell Peppers

Cooking Time: 30 minutes

Servings: 4

Ingredients:

- 4 bell peppers halved, and seeds removed.
- 1 cup cooked quinoa
- 1/2 lb ground turkey
- 1/2 cup tomato sauce (check for no onion and garlic)
- 1 teaspoon dried oregano
- Salt and pepper to taste

Instructions:

1. Preheat the oven to 375°F (190°C).
2. In a skillet, cook ground turkey until browned.
3. Mix cooked quinoa, browned turkey, tomato sauce, oregano, salt, and pepper.
4. Stuff bell peppers with the mixture.
5. Bake for 20-25 minutes or until peppers are tender.

Nutritional Information (per serving):

Calories: 300, Protein: 20g, Carbohydrates: 30g, Fat: 10g

Baked Chicken Parmesan

Cooking Time: 30 minutes

Servings: 4

Ingredients:

- 4 boneless, skinless chicken breasts
- 1 cup gluten-free breadcrumbs
- 1/2 cup grated Parmesan cheese
- 1 cup low FODMAP marinara sauce
- 1 cup lactose-free mozzarella cheese, shredded.
- Fresh basil for garnish

Instructions:

1. Preheat the oven to 400°F (200°C).
2. Mix breadcrumbs and grated Parmesan in a shallow dish.
3. Dip each chicken breast into the breadcrumb mixture, coating both sides.
4. Place the coated chicken in a baking dish.
5. Top each breast with marinara sauce and mozzarella.
6. Bake for 25-30 minutes or until chicken is cooked through.
7. Garnish with fresh basil before serving.

Nutritional Information (per serving):

Calories: 400, Protein: 35g, Carbohydrates: 20g, Fat: 18g

Salmon and Spinach Foil Packets

Cooking Time: 20 minutes

Servings: 2

Ingredients:

- 2 salmon fillets
- 2 cups baby spinach
- 1 lemon, sliced.
- 2 tablespoons olive oil
- 1 teaspoon dill, dried
- Salt and pepper to taste

Instructions:

1. Preheat the oven to 400°F (200°C).
2. Place each salmon fillet on a piece of foil.
3. Top with baby spinach, lemon slices, olive oil, dill, salt, and pepper.
4. Fold the foil to create a packet.
5. Bake for 15-20 minutes or until salmon is cooked through.

Nutritional Information (per serving):

Calories: 350, Protein: 30g, Carbohydrates: 5g, Fat: 22g

Tomato Basil Grilled Chicken

Cooking Time: 20 minutes

Servings: 4

Ingredients:

- 4 boneless, skinless chicken breasts
- 2 cups cherry tomatoes, halved.
- 1/4 cup fresh basil, chopped.
- 2 tablespoons balsamic vinegar
- 2 tablespoons olive oil
- Salt and pepper to taste

Instructions:

1. Preheat the grill to medium-high heat.
2. Season chicken breasts with salt and pepper.
3. In a bowl, mix cherry tomatoes, fresh basil, balsamic vinegar, and olive oil.
4. Grill chicken for 6-8 minutes per side or until fully cooked.
5. Top grilled chicken with the tomato basil mixture before serving.

Nutritional Information (per serving):

Calories: 300, Protein: 35g, Carbohydrates: 8g, Fat: 15g

Eggplant Lasagna

Cooking Time: 45 minutes

Servings: 4

Ingredients:

- 1 large eggplant, sliced
- 1 lb ground turkey
- 2 cups low FODMAP marinara sauce
- 1 cup lactose-free ricotta cheese
- 1 cup lactose-free mozzarella cheese, shredded
- 1/4 cup grated Parmesan cheese
- Fresh basil for garnish

Instructions:

1. Preheat the oven to 375°F (190°C).
2. Grill or roast eggplant slices until tender.
3. In a skillet, cook ground turkey until browned.
4. In a baking dish, layer eggplant, ground turkey, marinara sauce, ricotta, and mozzarella.
5. Repeat the layers and top with grated Parmesan.
6. Bake for 30-35 minutes or until bubbly and golden.
7. Garnish with fresh basil before serving.

Nutritional Information (per serving):

Calories: 400, Protein: 30g, Carbohydrates: 15g, Fat: 25g

Cilantro Lime Shrimp and Rice Bowl

Cooking Time: 25 minutes

Servings: 2

Ingredients:

- 1 cup jasmine rice, cooked.
- 1/2 lb shrimp, peeled and deveined.
- 2 tablespoons fresh cilantro, chopped.
- 1 lime, juiced.
- 2 tablespoons olive oil
- Salt and pepper to taste
- Sliced green onions for garnish.

Instructions:

1. Cook jasmine rice according to package instructions.
2. In a pan, sauté shrimp in olive oil until pink and opaque.
3. Mix cooked rice, chopped cilantro, lime juice, salt, and pepper.
4. Serve shrimp over the cilantro lime rice.
5. Garnish with sliced green onions.

Nutritional Information (per serving):

Calories: 350, Protein: 20g, Carbohydrates: 45g, Fat: 12g

CHAPTER 4

SNACK ATTACK: GUILT-FREE MUNCHING

Parmesan Rosemary Popcorn

Cooking Time: 5 minutes

Servings: 2

Ingredients:

- 1/2 cup popcorn kernels
- 2 tablespoons olive oil
- 1/4 cup Parmesan cheese, grated
- 1 teaspoon dried rosemary
- Salt to taste

Instructions:

1. Pop the popcorn kernels according to package instructions.
2. Drizzle olive oil over the popped popcorn.
3. Sprinkle grated Parmesan, dried rosemary, and salt.
4. Toss to combine and enjoy!

Nutritional Information (per serving):

Calories: 200, Protein: 5g, Carbohydrates: 20g, Fat: 12g

Cucumber and Hummus Bites

Prep Time: 10 minutes

Servings: 2

Ingredients:

- 1 cucumber, sliced.
- 1/2 cup low FODMAP hummus
- Cherry tomatoes for topping
- Fresh basil leaves for garnish.

Instructions:

1. Slice the cucumber into rounds.
2. Top each cucumber slice with a small dollop of hummus.
3. Garnish with cherry tomatoes and fresh basil leaves.

Nutritional Information (per serving):

Calories: 120, Protein: 5g, Carbohydrates: 10g, Fat: 7g

Strawberry Almond Energy Bites

Prep Time: 15 minutes

Servings: 4

Ingredients:

- 1 cup strawberries hulled and chopped.
- 1 cup almond flour
- 1/4 cup coconut oil, melted.
- 1 tablespoon chia seeds
- 1 teaspoon vanilla extract

Instructions:

1. In a food processor, blend strawberries until smooth.
2. In a bowl, mix strawberry puree, almond flour, melted coconut oil, chia seeds, and vanilla extract.
3. Roll into bite-sized balls and chill in the refrigerator.

Nutritional Information (per serving):

Calories: 180, Protein: 4g, Carbohydrates: 10g, Fat: 15g

Greek Yogurt and Berry Parfait

Prep Time: 5 minutes

Servings: 2

Ingredients:

- 1 cup lactose-free Greek yogurt
- 1/2 cup blueberries
- 1/2 cup strawberries, sliced.
- 2 tablespoons low FODMAP granola

Instructions:

1. In serving glasses, layer Greek yogurt, blueberries, strawberries, and granola.
2. Repeat the layers and enjoy.

Nutritional Information (per serving):

Calories: 200, Protein: 15g, Carbohydrates: 25g, Fat: 8g

Rice Cake with Peanut Butter and Banana Slices

Prep Time: 5 minutes

Servings: 1

Ingredients:

- 1 rice cake
- 2 tablespoons peanut butter
- 1/2 banana, sliced.

Instructions:

1. Spread peanut butter over the rice cake.
2. Top with banana slices.
3. Enjoy this quick and satisfying snack.

Nutritional Information:

Calories: 220, Protein: 6g, Carbohydrates: 25g, Fat: 12g

Roasted Red Pepper and Feta Dip

Cooking Time: 15 minutes

Servings: 4

Ingredients:

- 1 cup roasted red peppers, drained.
- 1/2 cup feta cheese, crumbled.
- 2 tablespoons olive oil
- 1 tablespoon fresh parsley, chopped.
- Carrot and cucumber stick for dipping.

Instructions:

1. In a food processor, blend roasted red peppers, feta cheese, olive oil, and fresh parsley until smooth.
2. Serve with carrot and cucumber sticks.

Nutritional Information (per serving):

Calories: 120, Protein: 4g, Carbohydrates: 5g, Fat: 10g

Dark Chocolate and Almond Clusters

Prep Time: 10 minutes

Servings: 4

Ingredients:

- 1/2 cup dark chocolate chips
- 1/2 cup almonds, chopped.
- Sea salt for sprinkling

Instructions:

1. Melt dark chocolate chips in a microwave-safe bowl.
2. Stir in chopped almonds.
3. Spoon clusters onto parchment paper and sprinkle with sea salt.
4. Allow it to cool and harden before serving.

Nutritional Information (per serving):

Calories: 150, Protein: 4g, Carbohydrates: 10g, Fat: 11g

Tomato Basil Bruschetta

Prep Time: 15 minutes

Servings: 4

Ingredients:

- 4 gluten-free baguette slices
- 1 cup cherry tomatoes, diced.
- 1 tablespoon fresh basil, chopped.
- 1 tablespoon olive oil
- Salt and pepper to taste

Instructions:

1. Toast gluten-free baguette slices.
2. In a bowl, mix diced cherry tomatoes, fresh basil, olive oil, salt, and pepper.
3. Spoon the tomato basil mixture onto the toasted baguette slices.

Nutritional Information (per serving):

Calories: 90, Protein: 2g, Carbohydrates: 10g, Fat: 5g

Carrot and Zucchini Muffins

Cooking Time: 20 minutes

Servings: 6

Ingredients:

- 1 cup grated carrots
- 1 cup grated zucchini
- 1 cup oat flour
- 1/2 cup almond flour
- 1/4 cup maple syrup
- 2 eggs
- 1 teaspoon baking powder

Instructions:

1. Preheat the oven to 350°F (175°C) and line a muffin tin.
2. In a bowl, mix grated carrots, grated zucchini, oat flour, almond flour, maple syrup, eggs, and baking powder.
3. Spoon the mixture into muffin cups and bake for 15-20 minutes.

Nutritional Information (per serving):

Calories: 150, Protein: 6g, Carbohydrates: 20g, Fat: 6g

Pineapple and Mint Salsa

Prep Time: 10 minutes

Servings: 4

Ingredients:

- 1 cup fresh pineapple, diced.
- 1/4 cup red bell pepper, diced.
- 2 tablespoons fresh mint, chopped.
- 1 tablespoon lime juice
- Gluten-free tortilla chips for dipping

Instructions:

1. In a bowl, mix diced pineapple, diced red bell pepper, chopped mint, and lime juice.
2. Serve with gluten-free tortilla chips for a refreshing salsa.

Nutritional Information (per serving):

Calories: 60, Protein: 1g, Carbohydrates: 15g, Fat: 0g

CHAPTER 5

DECADENT DESSERTS WITHOUT THE

DIGESTIVE DISTRESS

Chocolate Avocado Mousse

Prep Time: 10 minutes

Chilling Time: 1 hour

Servings: 4

Ingredients:

- 2 ripe avocados
- 1/4 cup cocoa powder
- 1/4 cup maple syrup
- 1 teaspoon vanilla extract
- Pinch of salt

Instructions:

1. In a blender, combine avocados, cocoa powder, maple syrup, vanilla extract, and a pinch of salt.
2. Blend until smooth and creamy.
3. Chill in the refrigerator for at least 1 hour before serving.

Nutritional Information (per serving):

Calories: 200, Protein: 3g, Carbohydrates: 15g, Fat: 15g

Berry Coconut Chia Pudding

Prep Time: 10 minutes

Chilling Time: 4 hours

Servings: 2

Ingredients:

- 1 cup lactose-free coconut milk
- 1/4 cup chia seeds
- 1/2 cup mixed berries (strawberries, blueberries, raspberries)
- 1 tablespoon maple syrup
- Shredded coconut for garnish

Instructions:

1. In a bowl, mix coconut milk, chia seeds, and maple syrup.
2. Let it sit in the refrigerator for at least 4 hours or overnight.
3. Before serving, top with mixed berries and shredded coconut.

Nutritional Information (per serving):

Calories: 180, Protein: 5g, Carbohydrates: 20g, Fat: 10g

Peanut Butter Banana Ice Cream

Prep Time: 5 minutes

Freezing Time: 4 hours

Servings: 2

Ingredients:

- 2 ripe bananas sliced and frozen.
- 2 tablespoons peanut butter
- 1/4 cup lactose-free milk
- Dark chocolate chips for topping

Instructions:

1. In a blender, combine frozen banana slices, peanut butter, and lactose-free milk.
2. Blend until smooth and creamy.
3. Freeze for an additional 4 hours.
4. Top with dark chocolate chips before serving.

Nutritional Information (per serving):

Calories: 220, Protein: 4g, Carbohydrates: 30g, Fat: 10g

Almond Flour Blueberry Muffins

Prep Time: 15 minutes

Baking Time: 20 minutes

Servings: 6

Ingredients:

- 1 cup almond flour
- 1/4 cup maple syrup
- 2 eggs
- 1/4 cup lactose-free milk
- 1 teaspoon baking powder
- 1/2 cup blueberries

Instructions:

1. Preheat the oven to 350°F (175°C) and line a muffin tin.
2. In a bowl, mix almond flour, maple syrup, eggs, lactose-free milk, and baking powder.
3. Gently fold in blueberries.
4. Spoon the batter into muffin cups and bake for 20 minutes.

Nutritional Information (per serving):

Calories: 180, Protein: 6g, Carbohydrates: 15g, Fat: 10g

Coconut and Lime Sorbet

Prep Time: 10 minutes

Churning Time: 25 minutes

Servings: 4

Ingredients:

- 1 can (14 oz) coconut milk
- 1/2 cup maple syrup
- Zest and juice of 2 limes
- Toasted coconut flakes for garnish

Instructions:

1. In a blender, combine coconut milk, maple syrup, lime zest, and lime juice.
2. Pour the mixture into an ice cream maker and churn for 25 minutes.
3. Transfer to a container and freeze until firm.
4. Garnish with toasted coconut flakes before serving.

Nutritional Information (per serving):

Calories: 220, Protein: 1g, Carbohydrates: 25g, Fat: 15g

Dark Chocolate-Dipped Strawberries

Prep Time: 15 minutes

Chilling Time: 30 minutes

Servings: 4

Ingredients:

- 1 cup dark chocolate chips
- 1 tablespoon coconut oil
- 1-pint strawberries, washed and dried

Instructions:

1. In a microwave-safe bowl, melt dark chocolate chips and coconut oil in 30-second intervals.
2. Dip each strawberry into the melted chocolate.
3. Place on a parchment-lined tray and chill for 30 minutes.

Nutritional Information (per serving):

Calories: 180, Protein: 2g, Carbohydrates: 20g, Fat: 12g

Lemon Almond Cake

Prep Time: 15 minutes

Baking Time: 30 minutes

Servings: 8

Ingredients:

- 1 cup almond flour
- 1/4 cup coconut flour
- 1/2 cup maple syrup
- 4 eggs
- Zest and juice of 2 lemons
- 1 teaspoon baking powder

Instructions:

1. Preheat the oven to 350°F (175°C) and grease a cake pan.
2. In a bowl, mix almond flour, coconut flour, maple syrup, eggs, lemon zest, lemon juice, and baking powder.
3. Pour the batter into the prepared pan and bake for 30 minutes.

Nutritional Information (per serving):

Calories: 220, Protein: 6g, Carbohydrates: 20g, Fat: 12g

Maple Pecan Banana Bread

Prep Time: 15 minutes

Baking Time: 45 minutes

Servings: 8

Ingredients:

- 2 ripe bananas, mashed.
- 1/2 cup maple syrup
- 2 eggs
- 1/4 cup coconut oil, melted.
- 1 cup oat flour
- 1/2 cup chopped pecans.
- 1 teaspoon baking powder

Instructions:

1. Preheat the oven to 350°F (175°C) and grease a loaf pan.
2. In a bowl, mix mashed bananas, maple syrup, eggs, melted coconut oil, oat flour, chopped pecans, and baking powder.
3. Pour the batter into the prepared pan and bake for 45 minutes.

Nutritional Information (per serving):

Calories: 250, Protein: 4g, Carbohydrates: 25g, Fat: 15g

Vanilla Coconut Chia Seed Pudding

Prep Time: 10 minutes

Chilling Time: 4 hours

Servings: 2

Ingredients:

- 1 cup lactose-free coconut milk
- 1/4 cup chia seeds
- 1 tablespoon maple syrup
- 1 teaspoon vanilla extract
- Fresh berries for topping

Instructions:

1. In a bowl, mix coconut milk, chia seeds, maple syrup, and vanilla extract.
2. Let it sit in the refrigerator for at least 4 hours or overnight.
3. Top with fresh berries before serving.

Nutritional Information (per serving):

Calories: 180, Protein: 4g, Carbohydrates: 20g, Fat: 10g

Cinnamon Baked Apples

Prep Time: 10 minutes

Baking Time: 30 minutes

Servings: 4

Ingredients:

- 4 apples cored and halved.
- 1/4 cup maple syrup
- 1 teaspoon ground cinnamon
- 1/4 cup chopped walnuts.

Instructions:

1. Preheat the oven to 375°F (190°C) and place apple halves in a baking dish.
2. Drizzle maple syrup over the apples.
3. Sprinkle ground cinnamon and chopped walnuts on top.
4. Bake for 30 minutes or until apples are tender.

Nutritional Information (per serving):

Calories: 180, Protein: 2g, Carbohydrates: 30g, Fat: 8g

CHAPTER 6
14-DAY MEAL PLAN

Day 1:

- Breakfast: Quinoa Breakfast Bowl
- Lunch: Greek Salad with Grilled Chicken
- Snack: Parmesan Rosemary Popcorn
- Dinner: Grilled Lemon Herb Chicken with Roasted Vegetables

Day 2:

- Breakfast: Cucumber and Hummus Bites
- Lunch: Low FODMAP Tuna Salad Stuffed Avocado
- Snack: Berry Coconut Chia Pudding
- Dinner: Baked Salmon with Dill and Lemon

Day 3:

- Breakfast: Chocolate Avocado Mousse
- Lunch: Mediterranean Quinoa Bowl
- Snack: Peanut Butter Banana Ice Cream
- Dinner: Low FODMAP Beef and Vegetable Stir-Fry

Day 4:

- Breakfast: Almond Flour Blueberry Muffins
- Lunch: Salmon and Spinach Foil Packets
- Snack: Dark Chocolate-Dipped Strawberries
- Dinner: Lemon Almond Cake

Day 5:

- Breakfast: Rice Cake with Peanut Butter and Banana Slices
- Lunch: Tomato Basil Grilled Chicken
- Snack: Coconut and Lime Sorbet
- Dinner: Eggplant Lasagna

Day 6:

- Breakfast: Berry Coconut Chia Pudding
- Lunch: Quinoa Stuffed Bell Peppers
- Snack: Roasted Red Pepper and Feta Dip
- Dinner: Baked Chicken Parmesan

Day 7:

- Breakfast: Vanilla Coconut Chia Seed Pudding
- Lunch: Tuna Salad Lettuce Wraps
- Snack: Maple Pecan Banana Bread
- Dinner: Cilantro Lime Shrimp and Rice Bowl

Day 8:

- Breakfast: Dark Chocolate-Dipped Strawberries
- Lunch: Greek Yogurt and Berry Parfait
- Snack: Lemon Almond Cake
- Dinner: Tomato Basil Grilled Chicken

Day 9:

- Breakfast: Cucumber and Hummus Bites
- Lunch: Quinoa Stuffed Bell Peppers
- Snack: Parmesan Rosemary Popcorn
- Dinner: Grilled Lemon Herb Chicken with Roasted Vegetables

Day 10:

- Breakfast: Chocolate Avocado Mousse
- Lunch: Greek Salad with Grilled Chicken
- Snack: Berry Coconut Chia Pudding
- Dinner: Baked Salmon with Dill and Lemon

Day 11:

- Breakfast: Almond Flour Blueberry Muffins
- Lunch: Tuna Salad Lettuce Wraps
- Snack: Coconut and Lime Sorbet
- Dinner: Low FODMAP Beef and Vegetable Stir-Fry

Day 12:

- Breakfast: Rice Cake with Peanut Butter and Banana Slices
- Lunch: Salmon and Spinach Foil Packets
- Snack: Dark Chocolate-Dipped Strawberries
- Dinner: Lemon Almond Cake

Day 13:

- Breakfast: Vanilla Coconut Chia Seed Pudding
- Lunch: Mediterranean Quinoa Bowl
- Snack: Roasted Red Pepper and Feta Dip
- Dinner: Baked Chicken Parmesan

Day 14:

- Breakfast: Quinoa Breakfast Bowl
- Lunch: Low FODMAP Tuna Salad Stuffed Avocado
- Snack: Peanut Butter Banana Ice Cream
- Dinner: Cilantro Lime Shrimp and Rice Bowl

CONCLUSION

As we reach the final chapter of "Low FODMAP Diet Cookbook for Beginners," I find myself reflecting on the profound connection between nourishment and well-being. This cookbook, born from the desire to ease a friend's pain, has evolved into a celebration of healing, resilience, and the transformative power of mindful eating.

Through these pages, we've explored the rich tapestry of flavors that can coalesce to create not just meals, but moments of joy and vitality. Each recipe is a testament to the idea that taking care of our bodies can be an act of self-love, and that the journey to a happy gut is a journey to a happier life.

As you navigate the culinary landscapes within, I encourage you to savor each bite with an awareness of the journey that brought this cookbook to life. Let these recipes be more than just instructions; let them be the companions that guide you towards a healthier, more vibrant version of yourself.

But our journey doesn't end here. Your feedback is the compass that will guide the next edition, the next chapter, and the next set of recipes. I invite you to share your experiences, your challenges, and your triumphs. Let your voice join the chorus of those who have discovered the transformative power of a Low FODMAP diet.

Did a particular recipe strike a chord with your taste buds? Did you find solace in the shared stories of those who have walked a similar path? Or perhaps you have suggestions for additions or modifications that could enhance the experience for future readers. Your insights are not just welcomed; they are integral to the ongoing narrative of this cookbook.

Reach out through the channels provided, whether it be email, social media, or our dedicated community forums. Let this cookbook be a cornerstone for the exchange of ideas, support, and shared victories. Together, we can create a community that extends beyond the pages of this book—a community bound by a commitment to health, happiness, and the joy of savoring each moment.

In closing, I extend my heartfelt gratitude for embarking on this journey with me. May the recipes within these pages continue to bring warmth to your kitchen, nourishment to your body, and a sense of connection to a community of kindred spirits. Here's to your deliciously happy life—a life crafted with intention, savored with gratitude, and shared with the world.

And so, until we meet again in the realms of delicious possibilities, happy cooking, happy eating, and most importantly, a happy, healthy you.

BONUS:

14 MINDFUL EATING GUIDE

Mindful eating is a practice that encourages a thoughtful and intentional approach to consuming food. By being present and fully engaged in the eating experience, you can foster a healthier relationship with food, promote better digestion, and enhance overall well-being. Here are some key principles to guide you in practicing mindful eating:

Eat with Awareness:

Before you start eating, take a moment to observe your food. Notice its colors, textures, and aromas. Engage your senses to build anticipation for the meal.

Eliminate Distractions:

Minimize distractions during meals. Turn off the TV, put away electronic devices, and create a calm environment. This allows you to focus on the act of eating and savor each bite.

Practice Gratitude:

Before taking the first bite, express gratitude for the nourishment in front of you. Reflect on the journey of your food from its source to your plate.

Chew Slowly and Thoroughly:

Chew each bite slowly and thoroughly. This not only aids digestion but also allows you to fully appreciate the flavors and textures of your food.

Listen to Your Body:

Pay attention to your body's hunger and fullness cues. Eat when you are hungry and stop when you are satisfied. Tune in to the signals your body is sending.

Engage Your Senses:

Use your senses to connect with your food. Notice the crunch of a fresh vegetable, the warmth of a soup, or the sweetness of a piece of fruit. This sensory experience enhances the pleasure of eating.

Appreciate Portion Sizes:

Be mindful of portion sizes. Serve yourself reasonable amounts and avoid the temptation to overeat. You can always go back for more if you are still hungry.

Check-in with Emotions:

Pay attention to your emotions and their connection to eating. Are you eating out of hunger or as a response to stress, boredom, or other emotions? Understanding these patterns can help you make conscious choices.

Mindful Meal Planning:

Plan your meals ahead of time. This helps you make healthier choices and reduces the likelihood of mindless snacking or reaching for convenience foods.

Express Mindful Gratitude:

After finishing your meal, take a moment to express gratitude for the nourishment and the experience. Reflect on how the food contributes to your well-being.

Practice Moderation:

Enjoy a variety of foods in moderation. Avoid labeling foods as "good" or "bad." Instead, focus on a balanced and varied diet that brings joy and nourishment.

Cultivate Awareness of Hunger and Fullness:

Rate your hunger on a scale from 1 to 10 before and after meals. This awareness helps you understand your body's signals and fosters a more intuitive approach to eating.

Experiment with Mindful Eating Techniques:

Try incorporating techniques like mindful breathing, where you take a few deep breaths before starting your meal or using mindful pauses between bites to assess your fullness.

Be Patient and Gentle with Yourself:

Mindful eating is a skill that takes time to develop. Be patient and compassionate with yourself as you cultivate this practice. Each meal is an opportunity to learn and grow.

Remember, mindful eating is about creating a positive and sustainable relationship with food. By adopting these principles, you can transform your eating habits, leading to a healthier and more enjoyable connection with the nourishment your body receives.